This manual is written for patients with bac[ ]participants in a back injury prevention progra[ ]who wants to have a healthy back.

— **H. [ ]**

SELF-HELP MANUAL

For Your Back

by H. Duane Saunders, M.S., P.T.

Published by
The Saunders Group, Inc.
4250 Norex Drive
Chaska MN 55318-3047

612-368-9214 or 800-654-8357
Fax: 800-375-1119

Table of Contents

Edited by *Robin Saunders*

Illustrated by *Mary Albury-Noyes*

ISBN Number 0-9616461-1-X

Back pain is no joke. It can be brought on by even simple movements, but with few exceptions, **back disorders are the accumulation of months or even years of poor posture, faulty body mechanics, stressful living and working habits, loss of flexibility and a general lack of physical fitness.** By middle age, almost everyone has felt some form of back pain; it is a potential problem for almost everyone at some point in his lifetime.

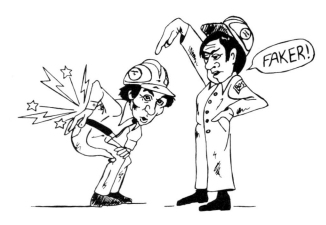

Back Pain Is No Joke

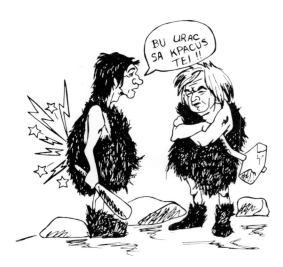

Back Injuries Are Not New

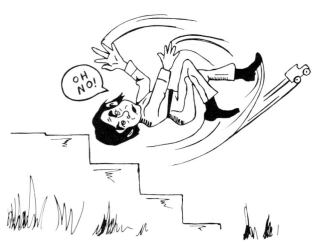

**Musculoskeletal Disorders are
Seldom Caused by a Single Traumatic Injury**

Back injuries are not new. Drawings on the walls of prehistoric caves show evidence of back injuries. Throughout history, the great numbers of people suffering back problems have produced innumerable treatments and quacks. Even since the advent of "modern medicine", some practitioners have attempted to group all people suffering from back problems into one category. Others have treated their patients with the approach popular with their "school of thought" rather than attempting to individualize programs.

Back problems are also incredibly costly. In business and industry, back disability is the top item in compensation payments and ranks second only to upper respiratory infections in payout for sickness benefits. It is estimated that 93 million work days may be lost each year because of back pain. Americans spend 17 billion dollars annually for diagnostic procedures and treatments, and additional billions of dollars on disability claims and lawsuit settlements.

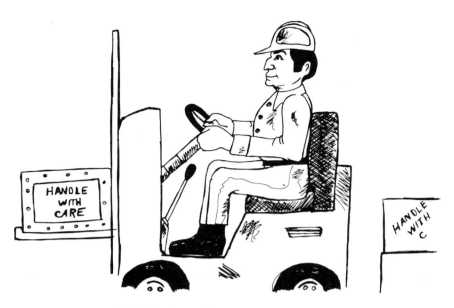

**Most back problems are unnecessary
and can be prevented.**

Back injuries seem to be difficult disabilities to cure and rehabilitate. A person who has had a backache is ten times more likely to have another backache than an individual who has never had a back problem. Many of our time-honored approaches to care and treatment of back problems have failed miserably.

The pain and expense of back problems is staggering and fundamentally unnecessary. Although there are no magic solutions, the answers to solve this dilemma are available. It is estimated that in the United States, 97% of the money spent for medical care is directed toward treatment of illness, injury and disability. Only 3% is spent on prevention.

It is time to take a new, fresh look at **prevention** of back injuries rather than face the frustration of **treating** them after they have occurred. Back problems can be prevented most of the time. Effective education is the key. Understanding what the problems are, how to prevent them and what to do if they do occur is the answer. It involves **self-responsibility** and a **desire** to have a healthy back.

Actually, there are some very simple things one can do to have a healthy back. In this manual you will learn why back problems are so common and read about recent changes in the way health care practitioners treat back problems. You will examine the principles of proper posture and will be shown the "power" position for the back. This is the position that should be maintained when sitting, standing, lifting or swinging a golf club.

You will be introduced to simple exercises that can be done to maintain the proper strength and flexibility necessary to live an active life free of back pain and you will learn many helpful hints for better back care.

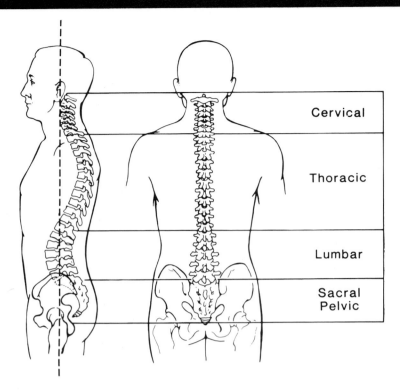

Our spine has to meet three definite purposes:

1. Maintain the structure of our trunk and allow for body mobility.

2. Protect the nervous system (spinal cord.)

3. Act as a shock absorber.

The bones (vertebrae), intervertebral discs and ligaments provide the structure. Muscles support this structure and joints provide mobility. The nervous system provides energy and control of the body.

The spine is not straight but is made up of four continuous curves. These curves allow for flexibility and help the spine in its role as a shock absorber.

Vertebrae and Facet Joints

The bones provide the structural support for your back. The *facet joints* control the amount and direction of movement.

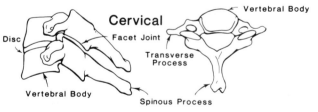

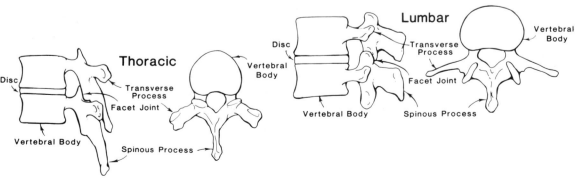

4

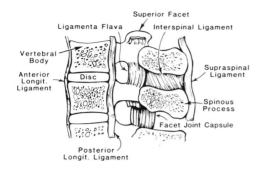

Ligaments

The *ligaments* are tough, non-elastic bands that hold the bones together.

Discs

The *discs* allow flexibility in your spine and act as shock absorbers. The center of the disc is jelly-like. It is surrounded by tough rubber-like bands that are attached to the bones (vertebral bodies.)

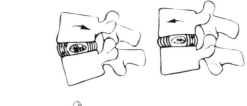

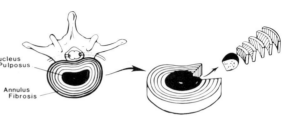

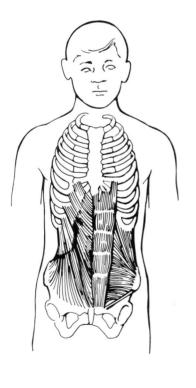

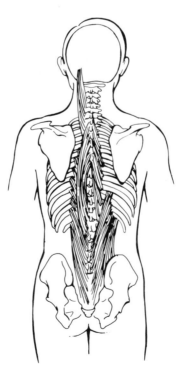

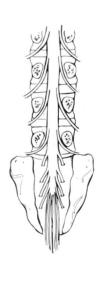

Muscles

The *muscles* contract to cause the body to move.

Nerves

The *nerves* provide the energy to make the muscles work.

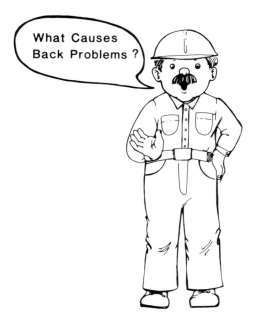

What Causes Back Problems ?

Back pain is rarely the result of one incident or injury. One of the keys to having a healthy back is understanding that most back injuries are the result of the cumulative effects of months or even years of poor posture, faulty body mechanics, stressful living and working habits, loss of flexibility and strength and a general lack of physical fitness. If you understand that things such as stooped posture, slumped sitting, improper lifting, twisting, weak abdominal muscles, tight hamstring muscles, emotional tension and even smoking can eventually lead to a back problem, it will become clear that changing some of these factors can prevent or even cure a back disorder.

Almost all back disorders are the result of:
1. Poor posture.
2. Faulty body mechanics.
3. Stressful living and working habits.
4. Loss of strength and flexibility.
5. General decline of physical fitness.

A back disorder begins to develop long before the first episode of pain is experienced and the problem is usually still there after the episode of pain subsides. The painful episode is usually caused by a simple twist, slip or even sneezing. Actually, this minor injury irritates the stiff and weak soft tissue structures in the back causing a painful episode of muscle spasm and inflammation. As the painful episode runs its course, the important treatment becomes preventing the next episode. So, prevention and treatment principles are really one and the same.

Poor Posture

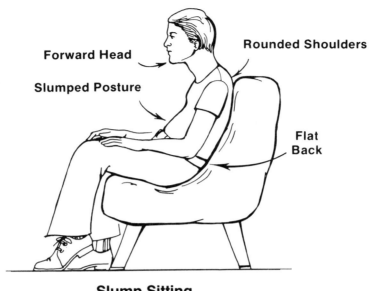

Forward Head

Slumped Posture

Rounded Shoulders

Flat Back

Slump Sitting

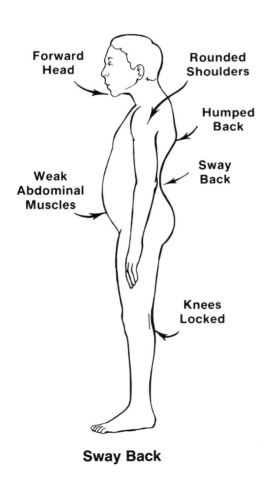

Forward Head

Rounded Shoulders

Humped Back

Sway Back

Weak Abdominal Muscles

Knees Locked

Sway Back

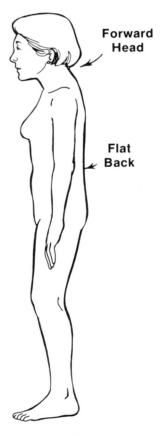

Forward Head

Flat Back

Flat Back

Common Causes of Back Problems

Faulty Body Mechanics

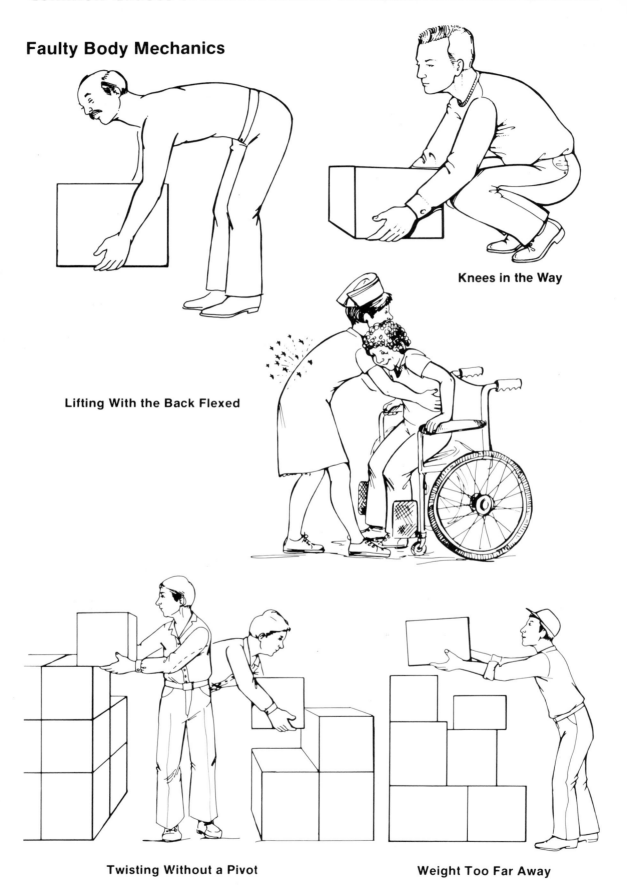

Knees in the Way

Lifting With the Back Flexed

Twisting Without a Pivot

Weight Too Far Away

Stressful Living and Working Habits

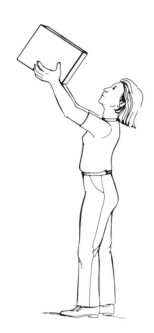

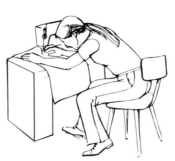

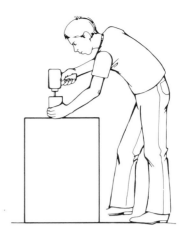

Work Too Low and Far Away

Reaching With a Heavy Load

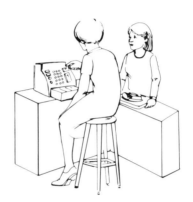

Back Unsupported

Poor Mattresses

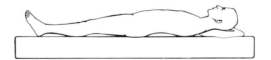

**A Mattress Which Is Too Hard
Leaves The Back Unsupported**

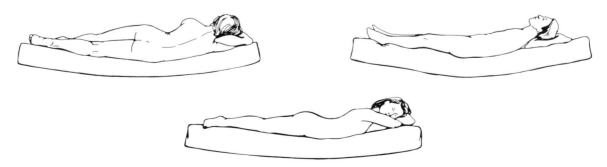

A Sagging Mattress Leaves The Back In An Unbalanced Position

Common Causes of Back Problems

Accidents

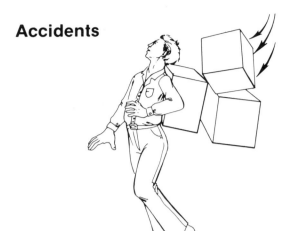

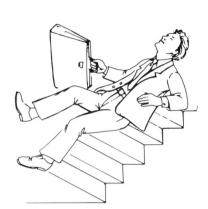

Loss of Flexibility

Decline of Physical Fitness

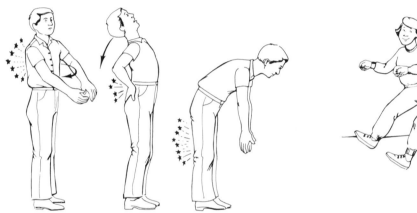

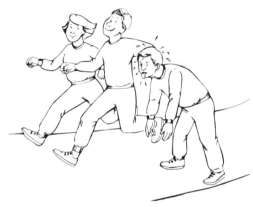

Other risk factors: Emotional stress, poor nutrition, lack of rest and smoking.

Remember . . . It is the cumulative effect of poor posture, faulty body mechanics, stressful living and working habits, loss of strength and flexibility and poor physical fitness that causes back problems. These are the RISK FACTORS of back injury. Eliminate them as often as you can and you will have a healthy back.

Uncommon Causes of Back Problems:

1. Birth defects.

2. Metabolic changes or problems.

3. Infection.

4. Tumors.

5. Psychosomatic problems.

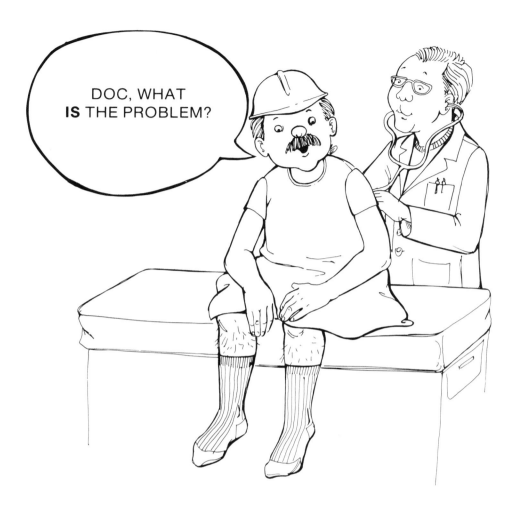

The most common back disorders are:

1. Muscle guarding and spasm.

2. Disc strain or bulge.

3. Disc herniation.

4. Acute strains and sprains.

5. Postural strains and sprains.

6. Joint stiffness.

7. Osteoarthritis.

**In this section, the cause,
pathology (description) and treatment
of these disorders will be discussed.**

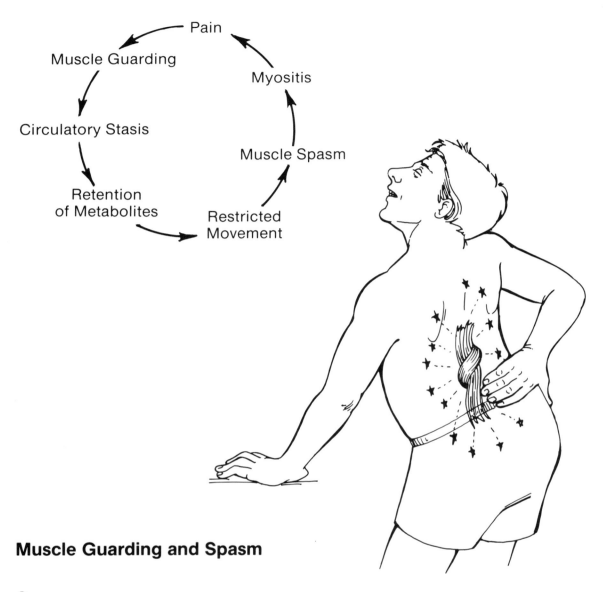

Pain → Muscle Guarding → Circulatory Stasis → Retention of Metabolites → Restricted Movement → Muscle Spasm → Myositis → Pain

Muscle Guarding and Spasm

Cause

Whenever you feel pain of any kind, your body's first reaction is muscle guarding. The muscles "splint" or immobilize the area where you feel the pain. Prolonged muscle guarding produces muscle spasm. Muscle spasm may be very painful but it is not necessarily a sign of a serious problem.

Pathology

Tender, painful muscle, slowed circulation and low-grade inflammation.

Treatment

The underlying reason for the muscle guarding should be examined and corrected to prevent recurrence. Ice packs, warm moist packs, warm baths, heating pads, muscle relaxant medications or just plain relaxation are sometimes necessary to relieve the problem.

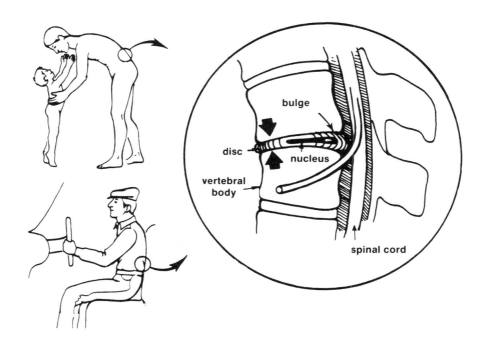

Disc Strain or Bulge

Cause

The two most common causes of a bulging disc are sitting or standing in a forward slumped position and forward bending and lifting. It is almost never the result of one injury and usually takes months or years to develop. Loss of flexibility and poor physical fitness are almost always related causes.

Pathology

The jelly-like center of the intervertebral disc is squeezed through the cartilage rings causing the outer wall of the disc to bulge. This puts pressure on the nerves in the disc wall which send back and leg pain messages to the brain.

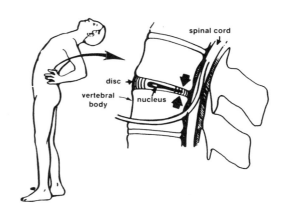

Treatment

There are probably as many "treatments" for bulging disc as there are for the common cold. Most of them are probably of no value and may even cause more harm to the disc. Proper treatment is correcting the faulty habits and posture which caused the problem. Backward bending flexibility must also be regained and proper balanced posture maintained until the disc has a chance to heal in its proper position.

In most cases, a small disc bulge can be prevented and/or corrected by backward bending and avoiding forward bending and slumped sitting for awhile. However, a word of caution: If this backward bending exercise causes increased *leg pain,* one should *stop.* Some *back pain* with this exercise is *ok.*

Disc Herniation
(Advanced Stage of Disc Strain or Bulge)

Cause

Slumped sitting, forward bending and lifting.

Pathology

Numbness, weakness, reflex changes in leg (for low back problems) or arm (for neck problems), as well as pain.

Treatment

Requires medical attention and physical therapy treatments such as traction. Severe cases may require surgery. Hopefully, this condition is recognized and managed when it is a small bulge and never gets to this stage.

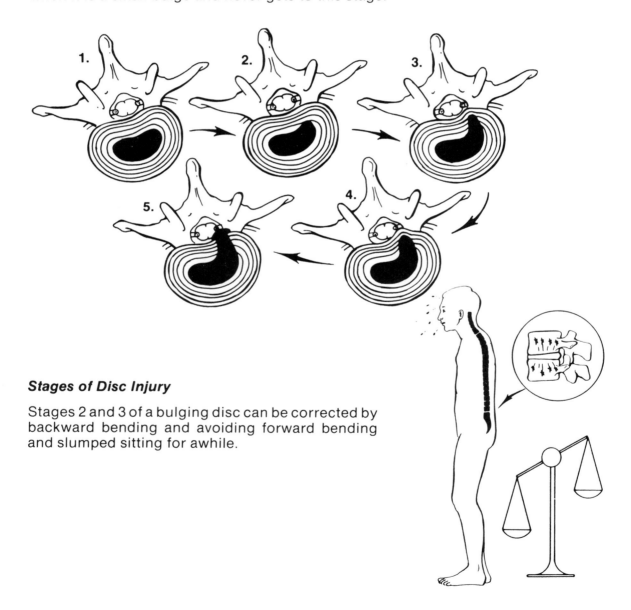

Stages of Disc Injury

Stages 2 and 3 of a bulging disc can be corrected by backward bending and avoiding forward bending and slumped sitting for awhile.

Acute Strains and Sprains

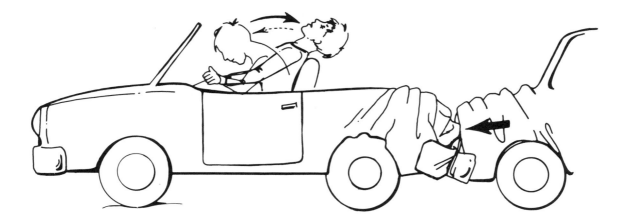

Cause

Improper lifting, twisting, falls or other injuries such as whiplash.

Pathology

There is often tearing, bleeding and/or irritation of the individual muscle or ligament fibers.

Treatment

If the injury is minor, a few days of rest and avoidance of further aggravation is usually satisfactory. If the injury is severe, considerable time may be required for healing. During the healing period, muscles will often become weaker, joints will stiffen and poor posture will develop. This resulting problem can be corrected with gradual reconditioning to restore full flexibility, strength and good posture. The help of a physical therapist may be necessary.

Postural Strains and Sprains

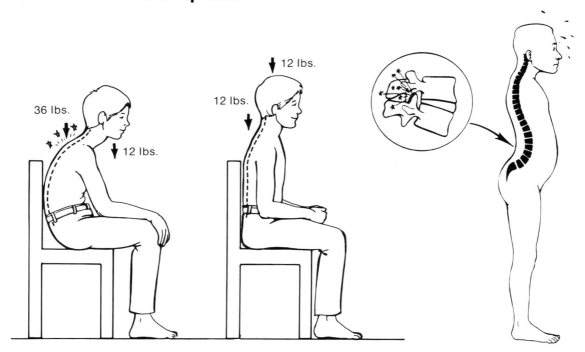

Cause

This problem is not the result of one injury or accident, but the result of many hours, days or even years of strain placed upon the joints and/or muscles because of poor posture and/or stressful living or working habits. For example, sitting at work or in a car in a slumped position, standing with the stomach muscles relaxed and the back in a swayed position for hours, or holding the head in a forward position too much of the time can cause this strain.

Pathology

Overstretching and/or irritation of the individual muscle and ligament fibers.

Treatment

General strengthening and flexibility exercises are helpful but most importantly, you should learn to correct the posture that is causing chronic pain. Changing positions frequently is helpful.

Joint Stiffness

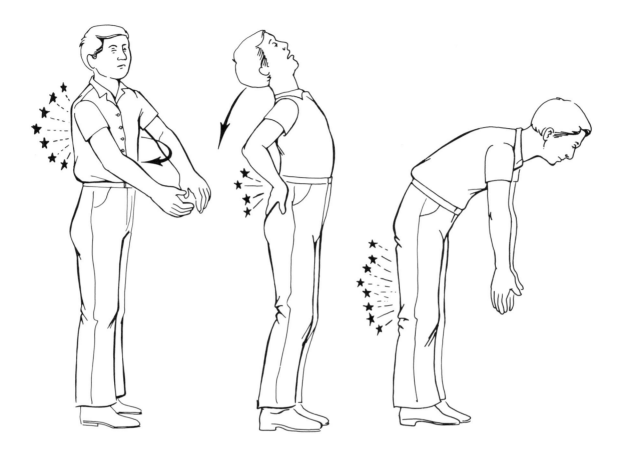

Cause

Stiffness may be the result of an acute sprain or strain healing without normal movement. It can also be the result of long-standing poor posture. For example, the person who always sits and stands with his back slumped in forward bending will eventually lose the ability to backward bend.

Pathology

The ligaments around the joints become thick and inflexible. When attempts are made to move the joint, pain results. The stiffness retards circulation to the joint, causing degeneration of the structures.

Treatment

Flexibility and stretching exercises and correction of faulty posture are the main things one can do to treat joint stiffness. Severe cases may require physical therapy such as ultrasound and traction.

Osteoarthritis

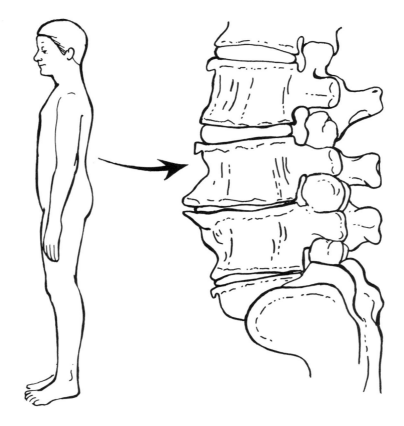

Cause

Osteoarthritis sometimes occurs as the end result of long-standing back disorders related to disc injury, strains or sprains or to repeated wear and tear.

Pathology

The description of osteoarthritis includes wearing out and narrowing of the disc and disc space, wearing out and roughening of the joint surfaces, thickening of the joint capsule and ligaments and narrowing of the intervertebral foramen (the space where the nerve leaves the spinal column.) The disc material may be absorbed by the body.

Treatment

Even though osteoarthritis seems serious and could cause many problems, we know that some people who have it actually have very little pain or discomfort. We also know that the incidence and severity of back pain becomes less as a person gets older (after 50-60 years of age.)

People who have osteoarthritis in their backs should exercise regularly because those who maintain a reasonable level of physical fitness and flexibility have less of a problem with osteoarthritis. On the other hand, overexertion and certain physically stressful activities may aggravate the condition and one should learn to avoid circumstances that cause significant discomfort.

Other much less common back disorders include:

Facet joint locking

The joints catch and lock in one position.

Joint instability

Can result from overstretching or torn ligaments (as in whiplash.)

Traumatic fractures

Rare, but serious result of an accident (a broken vertebra.)

Stress fractures

Very rarely occur as a result of repeated stress on the spine.

Compression fractures

Occur in older people (especially women) as a result of inactivity and metabolic changes.

Tumors

Very rare; may occur in someone who has had previous cancer.

Sacroiliac sprain

Usually results from heavy lifting, twisting, falling or pregnancy.

Coccyx fracture or sprain

Usually a result of a fall or direct blow to the tail bone.

Inflammation

Can occur in muscles, joints or disc, usually secondary to injury or aggravation. Inflammation is present to a certain degree with most of the other problems described earlier.

Disease and illness elsewhere in the body

Sometimes such things as kidney or prostate infections or meningitis cause back pain.

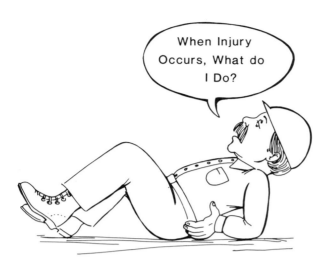

A great deal has been learned about back pain and back injuries in the past few years. For many years, most doctors and therapists treated individuals with back problems with passive treatments such as bed rest, medication, heat or cold packs and/or various forms of manipulation and massage. When these treatments failed, surgery often seemed to be the only thing left to do. All too often, in the end, the patient still suffered with back pain. It seemed that when a back injury occurred, the treatments helped in the short term, but in the long term, the problem kept coming back. In fact, it often became worse over time.

Many individuals with back disorders become more and more dependent upon treatment and more protective and inactive because it hurts to move. Being afraid to move causes them to become stiffer and weaker which of course makes the problem worse. Thus, a vicious cycle.

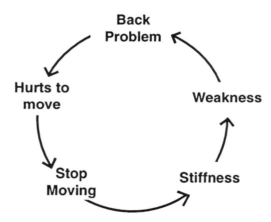

People with back problems often seem to be faced with this vicious cycle.

Today, all of this is changing. Considerable evidence now exists that bed rest and the various forms of passive treatment are at best of limited value, and at worst can actually be harmful. We now know that careful activity and the right kind of exercise is an important part of the treatment of back pain. In most cases, it is very important to start exercise and activity early, usually within a day or two after pain is experienced. This is true even when it is somewhat painful and uncomfortable to start moving. Or better yet, regular exercise, a healthy life-style and attention to proper body mechanics can be preventative as well.

Balance is the Key

Another key to having a healthy back is maintaining good balance in your spine as much of the time as possible. The human spine supports weight like a pillar, unlike the four-legged animal's spine which supports weight like a beam. Every time we stand or sit up, our backs must work against gravity to support a top-heavy structure. The normal spine has four gentle, continuous curves that help absorb shock and provide flexibility. The natural curves in your back allow weight to be shared by various structures in the spine.

If you have a sway back, flattened back, rounded shoulders or forward head, or if you spend long periods of time in stressful positions, your spine is not in its normal balance. This can either place a strain on the ligaments or cause excessive wear on some portions of the spine.

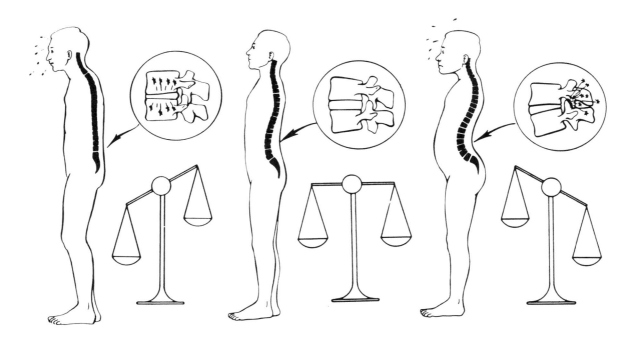

Immediate care:

1. Ice (If trauma has occurred.)
2. Rest from aggravation.
3. See your doctor/therapist.
4. Assume good posture.

As you improve:

1. Start moving.
2. Exercise carefully.
3. Recondition yourself.
4. Examine the incident.
5. Review back care.
6. Restore flexibility and strength.
7. **Maintain a balanced posture.**

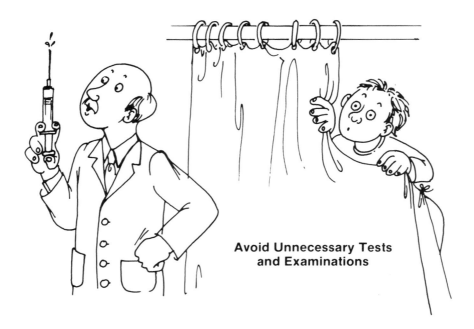

**Avoid Unnecessary Tests
and Examinations**

Evaluation — The Exam

Most physicians and therapists go through most of the steps mentioned here. Shortcuts must be avoided, but it is important to remember that each examiner will do things a little differently.

1. A complete history, which will frequently include the following questions: How did your pain first start? What was the exact position you were in when you were injured? What is the exact location of your pain? Does coughing or sneezing make it worse? What makes it better? What previous treatment have you received?

2. Physical examination to determine the following: Your general posture, muscle tone and range of motion; areas of local tenderness and muscle spasm; and possible muscular weakness and sensory changes in the extremities. A general abdominal, rectal and pelvic exam may be included to be sure there are no problems related to your back.

3. A physician may also want to use special studies such as laboratory tests, x-rays, myelograms and CAT/MRI scans to identify the extent of a disc problem or an electromyogram to identify nerve damage caused by a "pinched nerve". Although these tests are sometimes needed, in most cases they are unnecessary and should only be done when a severe problem is suspected or when standard, more conservative treatment doesn't seem to be helping.

Treatment of Back and Neck Problems

1. *Elimination of the cause*

The most important aspect of treatment in almost all cases is improving your physical strength, flexibility and fitness and correcting the poor posture and/or faulty working and living habits that caused the problem in the first place. You may need help from a physical therapist or a physician, but *you cannot expect to be cured without your willingness to assume most of the responsibility.*

2. *Posture correction*

It is essential that you assume and maintain a balanced, neutral lower back posture as soon as possible when back pain is experienced. Your body is trying to heal itself, but it cannot as long as poor posture positions are maintained.

3. *Back supports and pillows*

Back supports can increase intra-abdominal pressure which, in turn, unloads the spine by approximately 25%. This may allow you to assume correct posture and relieve pain so you can become active sooner. A lumbar pillow designed to support the neutral inward curve of the lower back while sitting is important, too.

4. *Medication, modalities and manipulation*

Medication, ice, heat, ultrasound, electrical stimulation, massage and manipulation are often effective in reducing pain, decreasing muscle spasm and increasing flexibility. However, they do not cure the problem.

5. *Rest and relaxation*

Rest from aggravating activities and positions is absolutely necessary for healing to occur. This does not mean that you must stop working and lie in bed, but you must remember to avoid those activities that aggravate your condition.

6. *Exercise*

Simple exercises can sometimes correct a back problem. General strengthening and flexibility exercises are extremely important in preventing back problems and play an important role in rehabilitation following injury. Unfortunately, certain exercise regimes have been recommended for people with "low back pain". These may be effective in treating some types of back problems, but they may make other types of problems worse. If you are experiencing acute back pain, an exercise program should be specifically designed for your problem. Follow the advice of your doctor or therapist.

Prevention of Back and Neck Problems

1. *Physical fitness and exercise*

   A regular (3 to 5 times a week) aerobic exercise program and good strength and flexibility are essential to maintaining a strong healthy back. Gradual conditioning is essential to prevent problems. It is not true that running or jogging is bad for your back. Any harm is usually caused from doing too much, too soon after a back injury. Good shoes are essential. Swimming is probably one of the best exercises you can do for your back if done regularly, but there are many other good exercises or sports that will keep you flexible and tone your abdominal and spinal muscles. See pages 35-48 for specific exercises.

2. *Practice good posture and body mechanics*

   Eliminating the cause of the problem is the key in both treatment and prevention and practicing good posture and body mechanics is one of the most important ways this is accomplished.

3. *Back support*

   A back support may be effective in reducing physical stress on the back when doing aggravating activities. It may also remind you to maintain better posture.

4. *Nutrition*

   Good nutrition is absolutely necessary for good health. If you are to avoid illness and injury, you cannot ignore this basic fact. Americans consume too many calories, eat too much sugar, salt and fat, especially saturated fats, and do not get enough fiber in their diets. Excess weight leads to increased wear and tear on the joints and can also cause poor posture, which contributes to back problems.

5. *Stress management*

   A tense person, more often than not, will have a backache. Flare-ups of back pain frequently occur at the peak or just after periods of increased tension. If you are willing to accept, understand and work to improve the emotional factors in your life, you will cope better with your back pain and improve your chances for a healthy back.

6. *Rest*

   Many clinical studies stress the importance of regular, adequate rest. You cannot expect to maintain good health if you ignore this important factor.

7. *Stop Smoking*

   Recent clinical studies show a direct relationship between smoking cigarettes and occurrence of back problems. Smoking restricts circulation and slows down healing when an injury occurs.

   In summary, think of your overall, total wellness as it affects, not only your back, but your health in general. It's your back and it's your responsibility to take care of it!

Posture — Sleeping

Sleeping on your stomach is not necessarily bad for you. There is no best position. You will probably find the one that's right for you.

What can I do to help my back ?

DON'T:

- Sleep on a sagging mattress. It puts the back in an unbalanced, stressful position and may cause a problem to develop.
- Sleep in one position too long, especially if sleeping for more than 7-9 hours.

DO:

- Sleep on a mattress that is firm, but not extremely hard.
- Waterbeds, properly adjusted, are satisfactory.
- A king or queen size bed allows freedom to change positions frequently.
- When getting out of bed, roll to one side and sit up sideways, using your arms to help.

Posture — Sitting

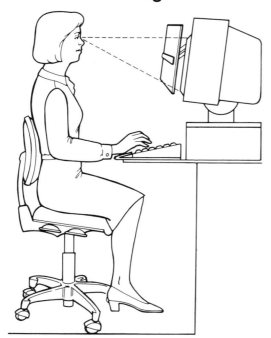 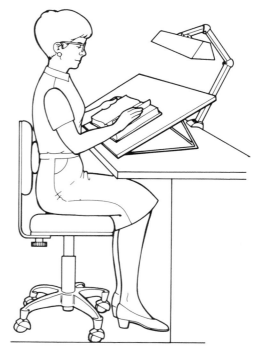

Sitting — Proper sitting posture is one of the best things you can do to prevent back and neck problems.

DON'T:

- Slump-sit (your low back should be supported.)
- Lean forward and downward to reach for or look at your work.
- Sit for long periods of time without getting up.

DO:

- Sit close to your work.
- Sit in a chair that is low enough to place both feet on the floor and no lower.
- Have a chair that supports your back in a slightly arched position.
- Maintain good sitting posture while driving. This frequently requires a small pillow against your lower back.
- Sit close enough to reach the pedals and wheel without slump-sitting.

What to look for in a chair:

1. Hydraulic controls
2. Seat back adjusts up/down
3. Seat back pivots forward/ backward
4. Seat pan tilts
5. Five caster-easy roll base
6. Seatback supports natural lumbar curve
7. Seat height adjusts
8. Waterfall seat front
9. Seat back and seat pan appropriate size for user

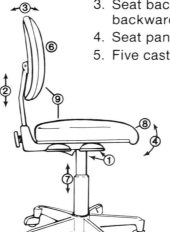

Additional features when needed:

- Arm rests
- Stool height with foot rests
- Self locking casters
- Material/fabric appropriate for environment
- Casters for carpeted versus vinyl floors.

Posture — Standing

Good balance is the primary goal.

DON'T:

- Wear high-heeled, hard heeled or platform shoes for long periods of time.
- Stand in one position too long.
- Stand with knees locked, stomach muscles relaxed, and swayed back.
- Stand bent forward at the waist or neck with your work in a low position.

DO:

- Elevate or incline the work surface for precision work.
- Put one foot up and change positions often when standing for long periods of time.
- Keep work up at a comfortable height.
- Change positions frequently.
- Stand on a cushioned mat.

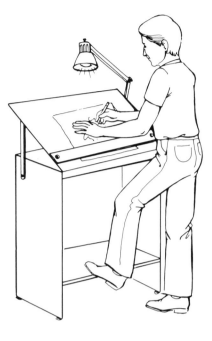

Work Height

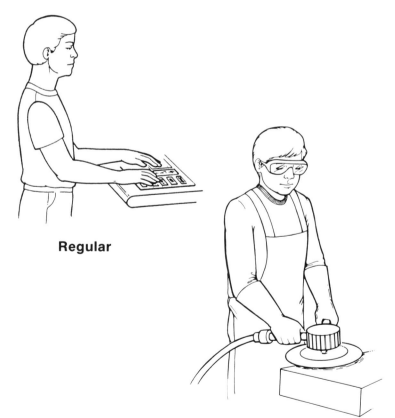

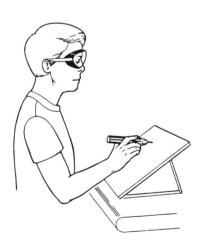

Light/Precision

Regular

Heavy

The "Power" Position

You now know that maintaining the neutral (slightly arched) position in the lower back is one of the keys to having a healthy back. It is important to maintain this neutral position when sitting or standing as well as when lifting objects or swinging a golf club. Athletes and coaches call it the "Power" position. To find the neutral position of the back, stand up straight. You should feel a slight inward curve in the lower back. Now, pull your stomach in and tuck your buttocks under. In this position you should feel the curve in your lower back disappear (flat back). Next, thrust your chest and stomach out to the front and stick your buttocks out to the rear. You will feel your lower back curve increase (sway back). It is undesirable to spend a lot of time in either the flat back or sway back postures. Now, return to the neutral (Power) position, which is actually somewhere between a stooped, flat back posture and the excessive swayback posture.

To bend fully backward and forward occasionally is fine; it helps you maintain good circulation and flexibility. Spending long periods of time in either position is stressful for your back, especially if you are twisting or lifting at the same time. For example, many golfers bend the back forward into the flat back posture when they swing. This is probably the number one reason so many golfers have back problems.

Once again, find your neutral position, then press your finger tips against your stomach muscles. As you do this, tighten your stomach muscles and make the front of your abdomen firm. Get the idea? Find your neutral position, then tighten your abdominal muscles to stabilize your lower back in this position. You should maintain this protective position for your back when lifting or when swinging a golf club. With practice, it is possible to maintain stability without feeling stiff or awkward. It is important to maintain this neutral position when sitting or standing, too.

You may need a back support or cushion to help you maintain good posture if you already have a back problem or spend a lot of time doing stressful activities. Can you find your neutral posture sitting? Remember, flat back — sway back — neutral, then stabilize.

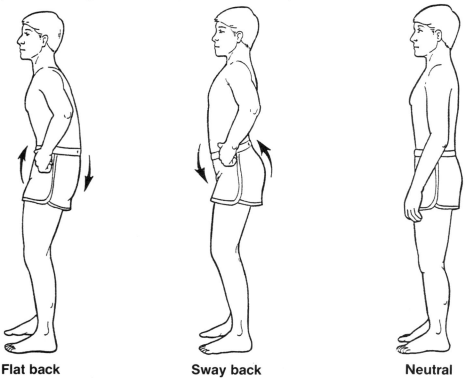

Flat back   **Sway back**   **Neutral**

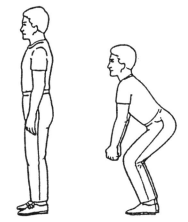

The "Power" Position

Now try this. Stand in the stabilized neutral posture. Bend your knees a little and bend forward but bend only at the hips — do not bend your back. It is helpful to think of keeping the chest and head upright. Keep the chest upright — don't bend at the back. This is the "Power" position; it is the secret to good body mechanics. Bend at the hips and knees, not the back.

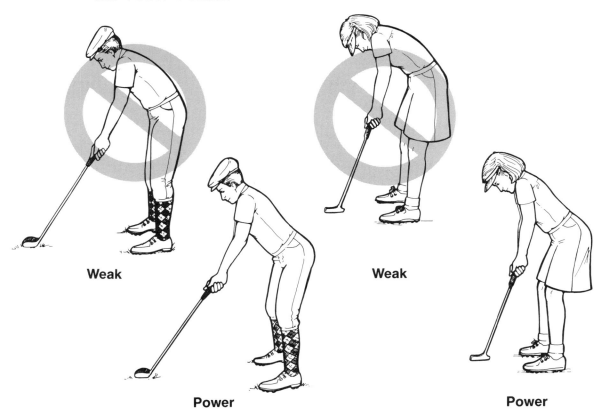

Weak

Power

Weak

Power

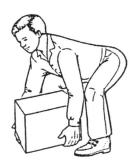

The "Power" Lift

If you are lifting something from the floor, the correct position is a lot like the three point stance of a football lineman. Bend the knees a little, the hips a lot, stick the rear out and keep the head and shoulders up. This is the three point stance position if you are playing football or it is the "Power" lift position if you are working at the factory. Even something as awkward as reaching into the trunk of your car can be done safely if you use the "Power" position.

Body Mechanics

Lifting, carrying and reaching — it's not how much you lift or carry, but how you do it. Here are some ways to use your body in the correct manner in work situations.

General Lifting Rules:

- Keep head high, chin tucked in and back in "power" position.

- Do as professional weight lifters do — keep back arched when lifting.

- Keep weight close to body and stand up straight.

- Use proper lift technique to get weight in close and maintain a wide, balanced base of support.

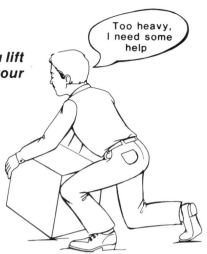

Plan Ahead
Test The Load Before Lifting

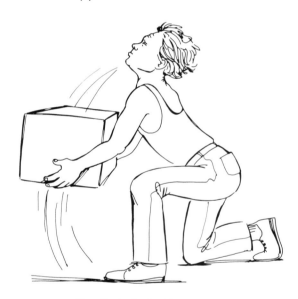

Don't Jerk As You Lift

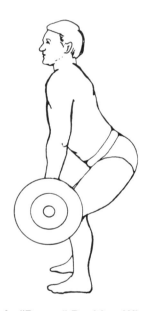

Keep Back in "Power" Position When Lifting
Keep Head and Shoulders Up

General Rules While Working:

- Clear your path.
- Keep feet apart for good balance.
- Wear comfortable, cushioned, non-slip shoes.
- Protect yourself.

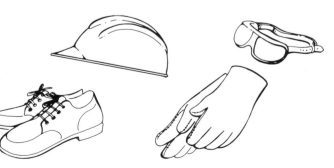

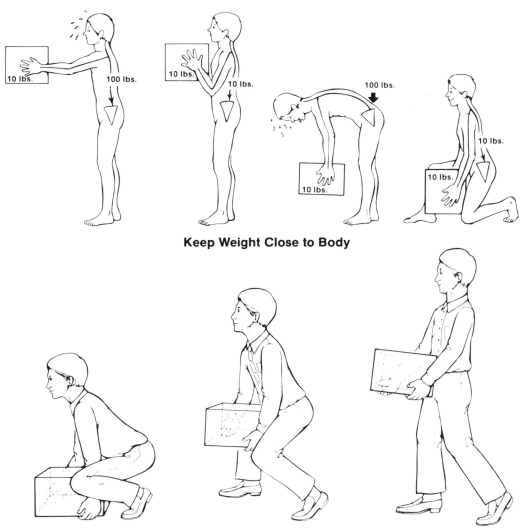

Keep Weight Close to Body

The Diagonal Lift
Squat, Head Up, Back Arched, Feet Spread One Foot Ahead As You Lift.

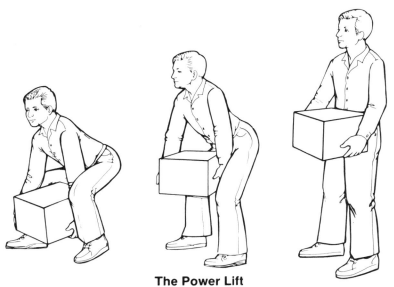

The Power Lift
Partial Squat, Head Up, Back Arched, Feet Spread One Foot Ahead As You Lift.

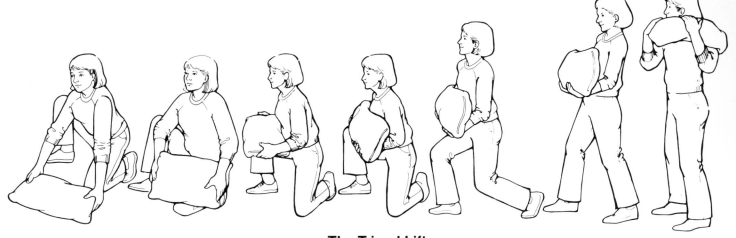

The Tripod Lift

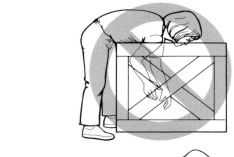

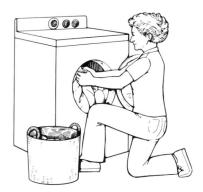

Kneel When Working in a Low Position

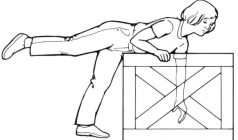

The Golfer's Lift

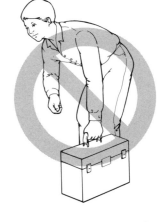

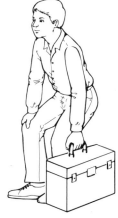

Partial Squat Lift

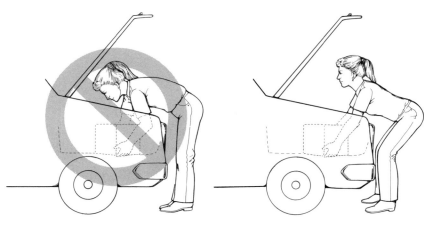

**Straight Leg Lift
Bend at the Hips, Not the Back**

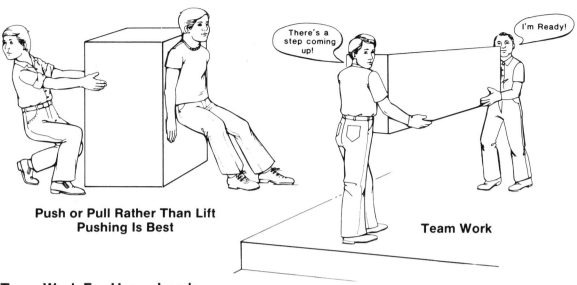

**Push or Pull Rather Than Lift
Pushing Is Best**

Team Work

Team Work For Heavy Loads

- Size up the load. Get help if it is too heavy.

- When two or more carry a load, one person should act as the leader. Be sure you can see where you are going.

- You can push twice as much as you can pull.

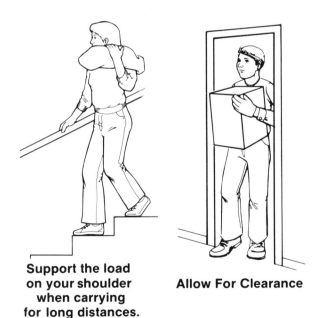

**Support the load
on your shoulder
when carrying
for long distances.**

Allow For Clearance

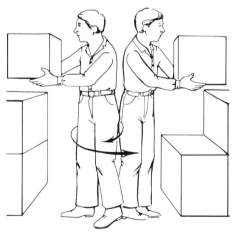

Pivot, Don't Twist

Other Important Tips

- Carry most of the load to the front.

- Pivot with your feet — don't twist!

- Allow for clearance.

DON'T

- Twist while lifting.

- Bend your back forward while lifting.

- Carry objects in a bent-over, stooped posture.

Interrupt or Change Stressful Positions Frequently

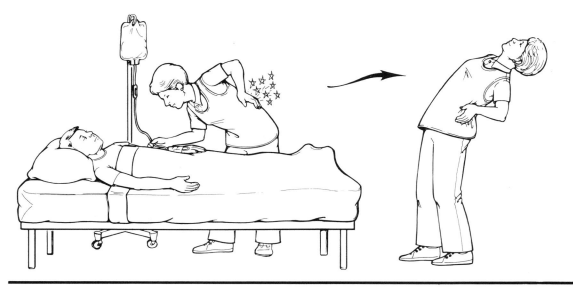

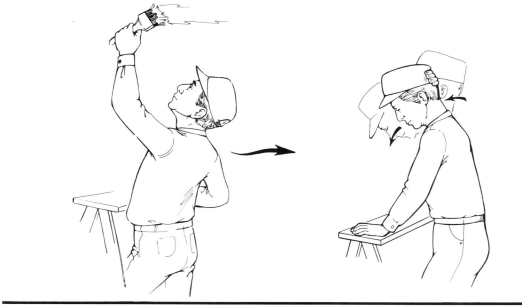

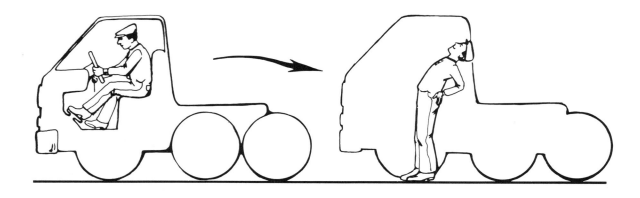

A Full Physical Fitness Program

We know that exercising regularly promotes cardiovascular fitness and reduces the risk of certain diseases. Exercise also promotes mental well-being. Many people exercise in order to look slim and trim, while others exercise to develop strength and flexibility to help them become better athletes.

While the list of reasons to exercise is a long one and you should not need further motivation, we want to give you one more reason. Exercise regularly so you can live your life free of neck and back pain.

There is considerable evidence to support the fact that regular exercise is the single most important thing that you can do to have a healthy neck and back.

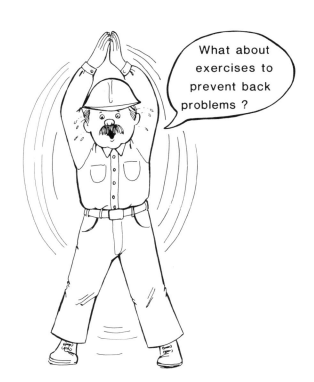

What about exercises to prevent back problems ?

Rules for Exercise

- Exercises should be done **regularly.**

- Always **start out mildly** and **increase gradually.**

- **A little pain with exercise is usually normal,** but **exercise should not cause pain that lingers after you have stopped exercising,** and exercises for the neck or back should not cause arm or leg pain.

There are four basic types of exercise:

- **aerobic**

- **strengthening**

- **flexibility**

- **relaxation**

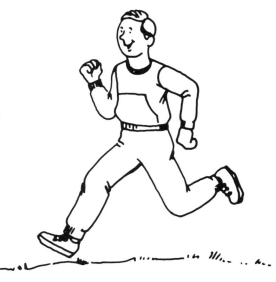

AEROBIC EXERCISES

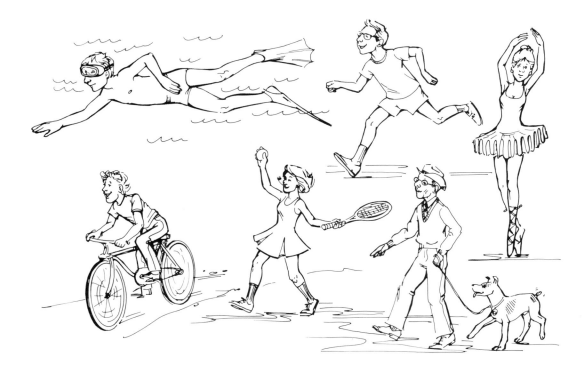

Aerobic exercises cause increased heart and lung activity and are done to improve cardiovascular fitness. Rhythmic, repetitive, dynamic activities such as running, bicycling, swimming, and walking that are sustained over a sufficiently long period of time, usually 20 to 30 minutes, are considered aerobic exercises.

Although one normally thinks of aerobic exercises as being beneficial for the heart and lungs, studies show that individuals who are in good cardiovascular shape are less likely to suffer from neck and back injuries. Therefore, the benefit of this type of exercise cannot be overlooked if you want to have a healthy neck and back.

Running, walking, swimming, bicycling and sports activities are all good for the back if approached in a common sense manner.

For an exercise to be aerobic, heart and breathing rate must be increased to an exercise level. As a general rule, a recommended exercise heart rate is $220 - \text{age} \times .7$. If you are 40 years old, that would be $220 - 40 = 180 \times .7 = 126$. Another way of judging if an activity is within the aerobic exercise range is to notice a definite increase in breathing rate but at the same time still be able to carry on a conversation without difficulty.

FLEXIBILITY EXERCISES

Earlier we learned that joint stiffness and loss of flexibility is a common cause of neck and back pain. Therefore, **flexibility exercises** are important for many. If a joint or muscle is stiff, pain will be felt at the limit of range of motion. This is not the case when a muscle or joint has normal flexibility. Therefore, one of the signs of joint or muscle stiffness is limited range of movement and pain at the end of the range.

"A good rule of thumb" is this: If you have limited movement and some stiffness is felt at the end of that movement, you will need to do flexibility exercises. If you seem to have full movement and no stiffness is felt, you probably do not need to do that particular flexibility exercise.

It is important to follow this rule because it is <u>possible to be too flexible.</u> Joints and muscles can be overstretched. Unfortunately, some athletes and exercise fanatics spend too much effort stretching. Weakened joints and muscles are the result. If you are not sure which exercises you should do, or how vigorous you should be, your physical therapist or doctor can advise you.

The following flexibility exercises for the neck and upper back should first be done as a test. If you feel stiffness as you do certain exercises, you will want to include these in your regular exercise program.

Forward head, slumped sitting posture involves rounding of the shoulders and upper back. The muscles and ligaments in the front of the chest and shoulders may become tight with this type of posture.

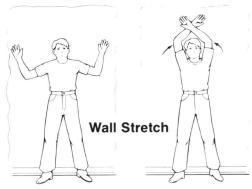

Wall Stretch

The wall stretch is done by standing with your back against the wall as you turn your arms out and raise overhead. Keep upper arms and body in contact with the wall as you do this exercise.

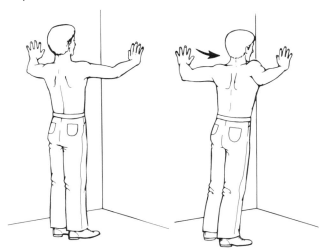

Corner Stretch

This exercise stretches the chest and shoulder muscles and ligaments. It should be held at least 15 to 20 seconds. Repeat the exercise a few times with hands at different heights until you feel you have gained flexibility.

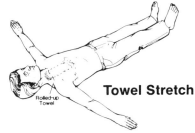

Towel Stretch

Rolled-up Towel

Another chest and shoulder stretch is done by lying over a towel roll as shown here. You may maintain this type of stretch for 3 to 5 minutes.

FLEXIBILITY EXERCISES

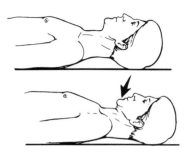

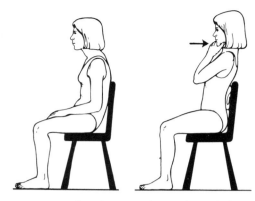

The head back, chin in, exercise is excellent for stretching tight muscles and ligaments in the back of the neck. Initially, the exercise can be done lying down, as shown . . . . .

. . . . . and advanced to the sitting or standing position as you make progress. If you work with your head and neck in a forward bent position it is good to do this exercise frequently to relieve stress and tension.

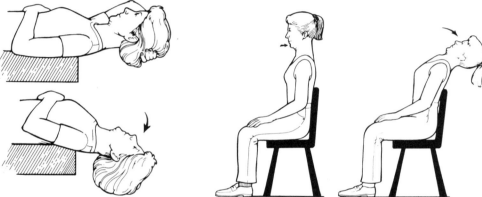

Backward Bending with Chin Tuck

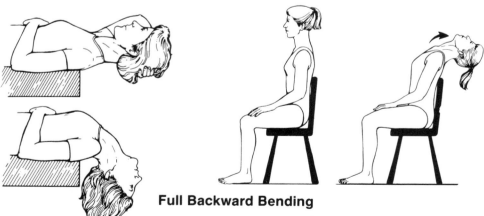

Full Backward Bending

Backward bending of the neck and upper back is especially helpful if you feel stiffness across the upper back and base of the neck. Start doing this exercise lying down as shown here, lowering the head slowly with your hand . . . . .

. . . . . and progress to the sitting position as you become more advanced. This is another excellent exercise for you to do frequently throughout the day if the forward bent head and neck position is a necessary part of your work. To concentrate the stretch to the upper back and lower neck, only do it with a chin tuck.

FLEXIBILITY EXERCISES

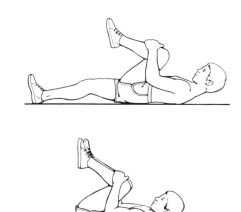

Exercises to Increase Forward Bending Flexibility — Lower Back

If you have an excess curve in your low back (sway back) and your back is stiff when you try to forward bend, you will benefit from exercises that stretch the low back muscles.

The exercises that stretch the lower back muscles are the single and double knee-to-chest exercises shown above on the right. Single knee-to-chest exercises are done alternately. You should hold ten to fifteen seconds with the knee flexed as close to the chest as possible. The double knee-to-chest exercise is also done with a five to ten second hold. One should do ten to fifteen of each of these as often as necessary to keep the back flexible. This exercise may aggravate a disc strain or bulge and should not be done if such a condition is present.

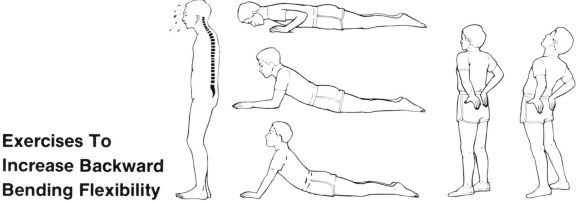

Exercises To Increase Backward Bending Flexibility

If you have a flat back or if you are stiff in backward bending because you stand and sit in a forward bent position or do a lot of forward bending and lifting, you will benefit from exercises that increase backward bending flexibility.

The exercises that increase backward bending flexibility are shown above. The press-up exercise is done by pushing up with the arms while the back and abdominal muscles are relaxed. This causes a passive stretch on the low back. The backward bending stretch is also done standing. These exercises should be done five to ten times each occasionally throughout the day, especially after you have been sitting or forward bending and lifting. These exercises would not benefit someone with a swayed back or someone with excess flexibility in backward bending.

FLEXIBILITY EXERCISES

Exercises To Increase Hip Flexor Flexibility

Tight hip flexor muscles and jobs that require a lot of standing can contribute to the sway back posture. They are sometimes caused by doing sit-up exercises incorrectly (feet stabilized while coming to a full sit up).

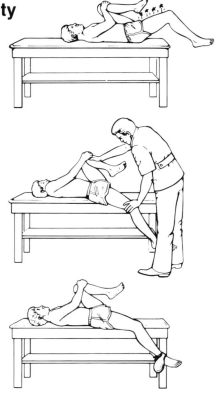

You should be able to lie on a table as shown above and bring one knee toward the chest until the lower back is flat while the opposite thigh remains on the table. You should also be able to bend your knee to at least 80° while in this position. If you cannot do this, you have tight hip flexor muscles. Tight hip flexor muscles may make the standing swayed back posture worse. Tight hip flexors can be stretched by using the methods shown. Hold each stretched position for several seconds, making sure the lower back is as flat as possible. Repeat this exercise several times a day.

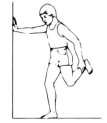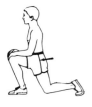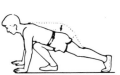

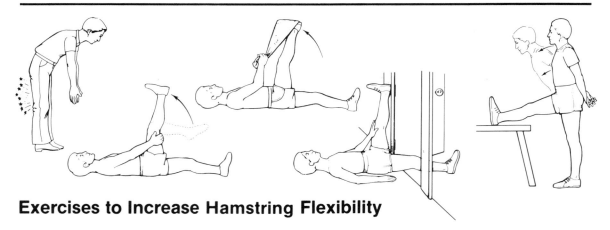

Exercises to Increase Hamstring Flexibility

Tight hamstring muscles prevent the pelvis from rolling forward as you forward bend; this will cause an increased stress on the low back. If you have tight hamstrings you will feel a pulling up the back of your thighs as you bend forward.

You should be able to extend your leg straight with your hip at a 90° angle while lying on your back as shown in this drawing. If you cannot do this you have tight hamstrings and should do this flexibility exercise. It is done as shown here. Simply hold the leg extended as straight as possible for five to ten seconds. Repeat the exercise five to ten times, one or two sessions per day.

40

FLEXIBILITY EXERCISES

Exercise to Increase Trunk Rotation Flexibility

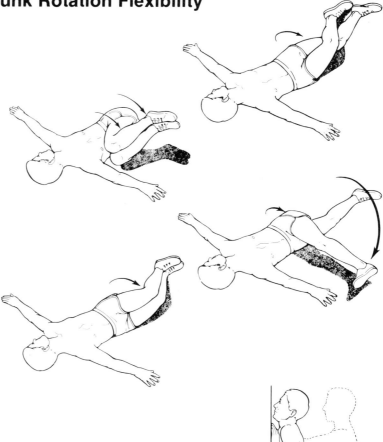

If your spine is stiff when you try to rotate or twist, you will benefit from these exercises.

If you flex the hips and knees and bring your thighs toward your chest when you do the rotation flexibility exercises, you will stretch the mid-back area. If you have your knees and hips bent with your feet on the floor, the stretch is more effective for the lower back area. If you raise one leg straight overhead or cross one over the other as you do the rotation exercise, you are doing a more advanced stretch. Note that the head is rotated to the opposite direction with all of these exercises. You should hold each stretch ten to fifteen seconds.

Exercise to Stretch the Calf Muscles and Heel Cords

If you have tightness of the heel cords or calf muscles, you will benefit from the exercise shown to the right.

Stand at arms length from the wall, keep your feet flat on the floor as you lean your body toward the wall. Hold each stretch ten to fifteen seconds.

Exercises to Stretch the Adductor (Inside Thigh) Muscles

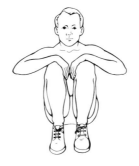
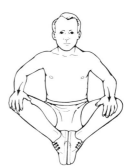

If your inside thigh muscles are tight, you will benefit from the exercise shown on the right. Sit with your feet braced together and spread your knees apart. You may apply additional force with your hands as shown. Hold each stretch position for ten to fifteen seconds.

STRENGTHENING EXERCISES

To maintain good posture and have a healthy back you must have good, well balanced muscular strength.

For strengthening exercises to be effective, the muscles must become fatigued while exercising. This increased work load causes the muscle to grow stronger. If your muscles are weak, only mild exercise will be needed to fatigue the muscle. As you grow stronger, more repetition or resistance must be added to work the muscle enough to make it grow even stronger.

Generally speaking, exercises utilizing heavy resistance and fewer repetitions build power, or muscle bulk, while exercising with mild resistance and greater repetitions build endurance.

Power is needed for heavy work activities and certain sports. Endurance is more important for good posture and most of our everyday working and living activities.

Resistance may be added to most exercises in the form of free weights, exercise machines or elastic stretch material such as rubber tubing. Sometimes just working against gravity is enough resistance.

Exercises to Strengthen the Neck

A very effective way to strengthen the neck muscles is with elastic tubing attached to a head band. The resistance can be varied from very light to very heavy depending on the size of the tubing and the tension applied. These exercises can be done in rotation, side bending, forward bending and backward bending.

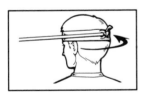 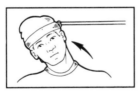 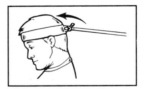 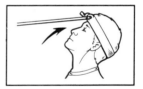

The head back, chin in, exercise that was shown earlier as a flexibility exercise, is also a strengthening exercise, especially if done against the resistance of gravity as shown below.

This side lying exercise is an especially effective neck strengthening exercise. A small pillow can be placed under the head to shorten the range of motion of this exercise if movement through full range of motion causes aggravation.

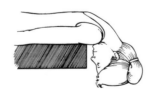

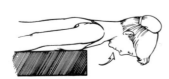

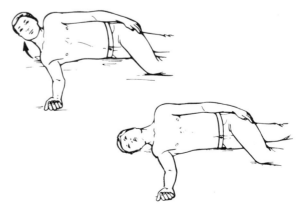

STRENGTHENING EXERCISES

Exercises for Strengthening the Upper Back and Shoulders

Chronic forward head posture, slumped sitting and round shoulders can cause stress on the joints and muscles in the upper back and neck. It is important to strengthen the neck and upper back muscles to correct this postural problem.

Strengthening exercises for forward head, slumped sitting and round shoulder posture and/or weakness of the muscles in the neck, upper back and shoulders are shown below. These exercises should be done once or twice daily, starting with a few of each and gradually increasing the number as tolerated. The back strengthening exercises shown on page 46 will also benefit.

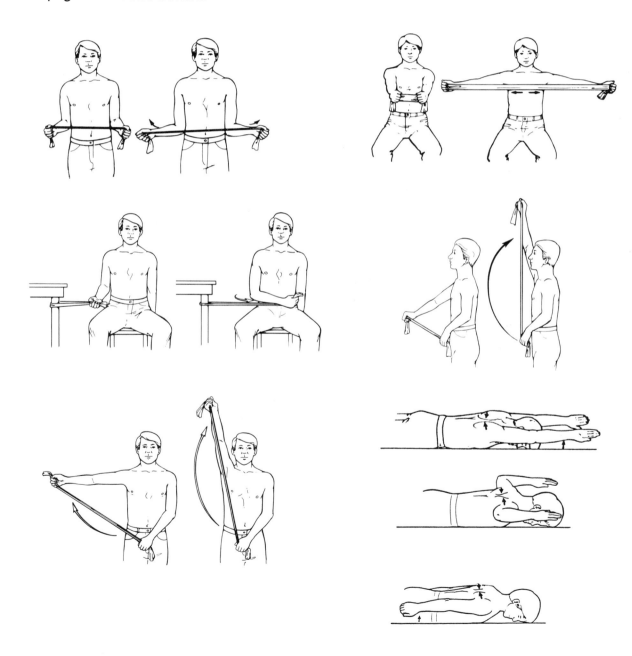

43

STRENGTHENING EXERCISES

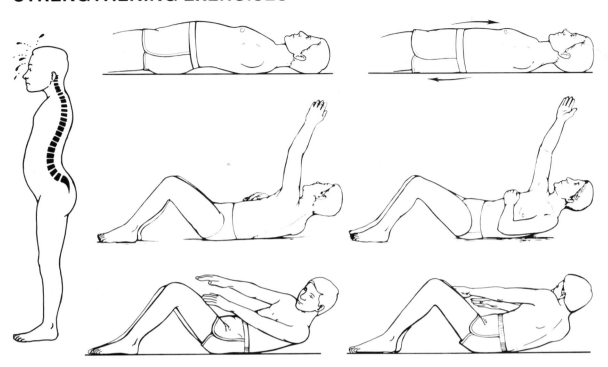

Exercises For Strengthening Abdominal Muscles

Weak abdominal muscles, jobs that require a lot of standing, pregnancy, and obesity (large protruding abdomen) sometimes contribute to sway back posture.

The pelvic tilt exercise will help strengthen your abdominal muscles as well as help reduce the curve in your lower back if you have sway back.

The pelvic tilt is done by tightening the abdominal muscles and the buttocks muscles at the same time. This pulls the pelvis up and forward in the front and down and backward in the back. If you have sway back and weak abdominals, you should practice this exercise frequently both while lying down and while standing.

Partial situps are done to strengthen the abdominal muscles. It is important to have strong abdominal muscles because they help increase intra-abdominal pressure while lifting. This takes some of the weight bearing and stress off the spine.

Partial situps are done correctly with the hips and knees slightly bent. One should raise the arms, head and shoulders off the floor as shown. The position is held for five to ten seconds. One should never raise to the point that the lower back is lifted from the floor. This causes too much pressure on the disc and is unnecessary for abdominal muscle strengthening. The feet should not be stabilized; stabilizing the feet will allow the hip flexor muscles to do the work and you may be getting the opposite effect that you want with this exercise. It is important that the pelvis be tilted in order to keep the lower back flat on the floor throughout the exercise.

The partial situp should be done with a slight right and left twist to strengthen the oblique muscles of the abdomen. Strengthening exercises such as this should be started mildly and gradually increased in number as the muscles get stronger. They should be done once or twice a day. These exercises cause increased pressure on the disc and should not be done by someone with an active disc disorder.

44

STRENGTHENING EXERCISES

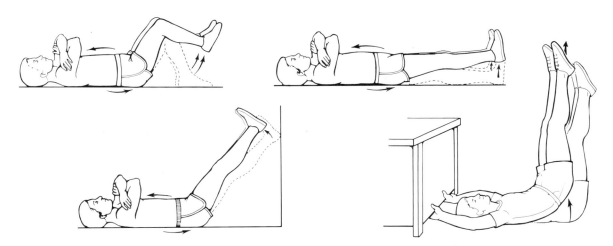

Exercises for Strengthening Abdominal Muscles

The double straight leg raise is an excellent exercise for strengthening the lower abdominals. The pelvic tilt (see page 44) is a necessary part of the double straight leg raise and must always be done while doing this exercise.

The double straight leg raise is done correctly by first doing a pelvic tilt to press your lower back against the floor, then raise the legs a few inches and hold 5 to 10 seconds. If you are unable to hold your lower back against the floor as you raise your legs, your abdominal muscles are weak and you should start this exercise with knees bent or with your feet against the wall as shown. As you become stronger, you can gradually advance toward the flat double straight leg raise or the double leg lift with the hips flexed. These are the most advanced ways to do this exercise.

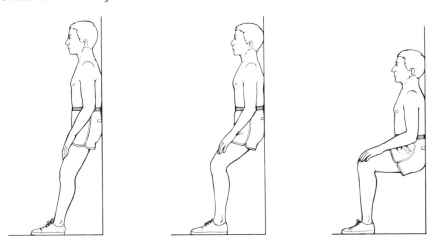

Exercises to Strengthen Quadricep Muscles

The quadricep muscles help extend the legs from the squat position. They are especially important if you do alot of lifting from the squat position. To strengthen the quadricep muscles, stand with your feet together approximately 18″ from the wall, lean against the wall and slide your back down the wall until your hips and knees are bent. Hold this position for fifteen to thirty seconds. If you are stronger, slide further until your hips and knees are at 90 degree angles. Also as you become stronger, the hold time can be increased.

STRENGTHENING EXERCISES

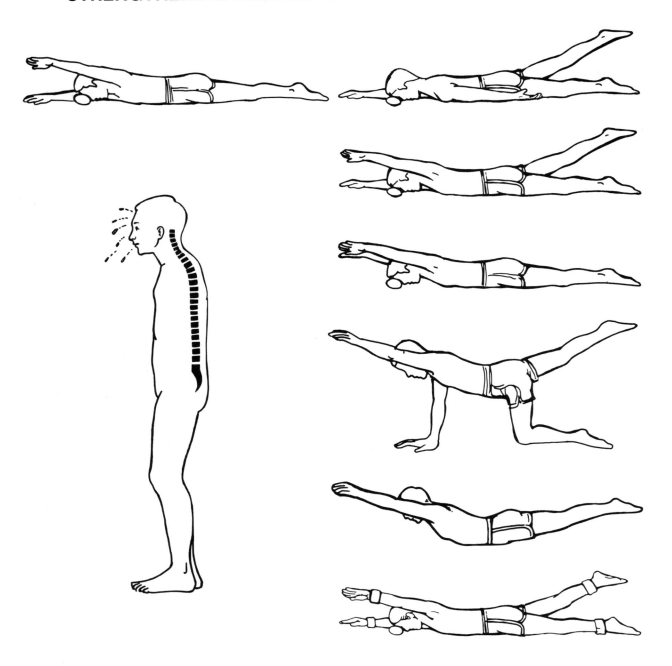

Exercises to Strengthen Back Muscles

Weak back muscles and jobs that require a lot of sitting or standing in the forward bent position often contribute to a flat back posture.

This drawing shows exercises that will strengthen your back muscles. If you do a lot of sitting or forward bending and lifting, these exercises will be especially beneficial. These exercises should be started gradually and done once or twice a day. You may increase to doing 40 to 50 each. Small ankle and wrist weights can be added to make these exercises more advanced.

RELAXATION EXERCISES

The following exercises are very helpful for any person who is tense and under stress or who has a job in which he must do a lot of sitting or standing throughout the day and does not have a chance to move or change positions frequently. They help to counteract the tendency to develop tight, sore muscles because of sitting or standing in undesirable postures. They should be done once an hour or whenever muscular tightness is noticed.

1. Close your eyes, relax your shoulders, then take ten deep breaths, breathing in through your nose and out through your mouth.

2. Circle your feet from the ankles —first together, then one at a time, twenty times each foot.

3. Lift your heels and press your toes into the floor, then lift your toes and press your heels into the floor. Repeat ten times for each foot.

4. With your arms at your sides, circle your shoulders forward ten times, then backward ten times.

5. If sitting in a chair, move back in the seat. Lift one buttock off the seat, feeling the muscles on both sides tighten as you do; hold while you count slowly to five; relax. Repeat for the other side. Now do the exercise three more times on each side.

6. Press your lower back into the seat, then arch forward ten times. Repeat ten times.

7. While sitting in a chair, press your knees and thighs together and tighten the buttock muscles; hold for five seconds; relax. Repeat four times.

8. Link your fingers together and place your arms behind your head with the elbows pointing forward. Gently push your head into your hands; hold for five seconds; relax. Repeat four times.

9. Slowly circle your head in one direction, then the other. Repeat ten times.

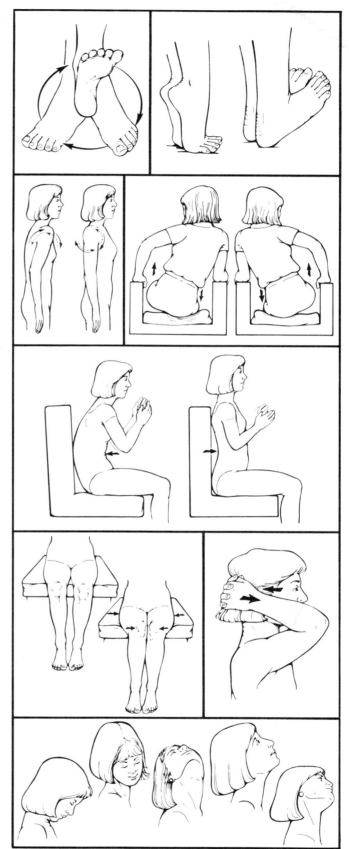

LAST WORDS!

It is true that many of us work hard at our jobs and it is sometimes difficult to think that we should exercise when we are already tired from work. However, you should remember that hard work and exercise are not always accomplishing the same thing. In most work situations, we get too much of one type of activity or exercise and usually not enough of another. Many people work hard all day yet are still very stiff and are in poor cardiovascular condition. An exercise program should emphasize the type of exercise that is lacking at work. For example, if one spends a lot of time flexing (forward bending) at work, he should emphasize extension (backward bending) exercises at home.